Beating Acute Myeloid Leukemia

A Cancer Survivor's Story

William D. Bramlett

Copyright

This memoir recalls the author's recent medical experience with cancer. It is not a substitute for professional medical or mental health advice. There are no references to the names of medical professionals. The author's family members have given permission for the use of their first names only.

Dedication

I dedicate this to the men and women who have invested entire careers searching for cancer cures. I also recognize and wholeheartedly thank the professionals who took me by the hand, leading me through my cancer journey. They are too numerous to mention by name:

Oncologists, Nurse Practitioners, Physicians Assistants, Registered Nurses and LPNs at Methodist Hospital and Frauenshuh Cancer Center, St. Louis Park, MN.

Oncologists, Bone Marrow Transplant Specialists, Radiologists, Nurse Practitioners, Physicians Assistants, Registered Nurses, LPNs, Dieticians and Physical Therapists at the University of Minnesota Hospital and Masonic Cancer Clinic, Minneapolis, MN.

With loving appreciation to my wife and caregiver, Diane, and my Minnesota family and extended family and friends around the country.

Special Dedication

Without a doubt, I would not be here except for the unselfish gift of stem cells I received from a young man from Germany.

Donors and recipients, through *Be The Match*, pledge to remain anonymous from each other until at least two years after transplant.

I look forward to communicating with my donor after February 2024, if he is willing.

His gift has humbled and possibly healed me from cancer.

Introduction

Everyone knows someone who has experienced the terror a bout with cancer brings. Most of us have friends or relatives who died from some form of the disease. But we are looking in from the outside until our first personal meeting with an oncologist.

I am one of those. Throughout life, I lost my father, a sister-in-law, aunts, uncles, cousins, and friends. My mom's mother died of bone cancer, possibly caused by the same leukemia I have fought. Dad lost his battle with stomach cancer, relatively young. Two favorite aunts fought breast cancer and lost, and a number of friends and co-workers died of pancreatic cancer.

But I failed to truly relate or understand until diagnosed with prostate cancer at sixty-nine.

I considered myself fortunate to live nearly seventy-years with nothing more than a broken nose, compliments of a teammate at high school football practice. No other broken bones, no stitches, no surgeries, no allergies, no hospital stays. Catching a cold was a rarity and other people caught the flu, not me.

Until prostate surgery, at age seventy, the meaning of the term in-patient escaped me. Intuitively, I understood it. I had heard about bad hospital food and the desire to get home to one's own bed.

The need for self-advocacy increases for the inpatient. At times, questioning the hospital staff is important. As is the willingness to trust their ultimate recommendations.

I have learned that inpatient means much more than a simple hospital stay.

My years of good health led me to state to friends and family a readiness to handle whatever might come after age seventy. Appreciating my life of avoiding doctors, I took a "bring it on" attitude. That was a mistake.

An old adage is, "Be careful what you say."

It is now two and a half years since the good doctors at Mayo Clinic, Rochester, MN., cured my prostate cancer. The experience prepared me well for my next cancer adventure, acute myeloid leukemia.

If cancer doesn't kill you, the disease changes your life forever. The goal of these chapters is to help anyone faced with the terrifying diagnosis of AML or cancer in general.

I do not intend to mislead anyone with my title, *Beating Acute Myeloid Leukemia*. The odds against survival are poor and difficult to accept. But beating the disease is possible, both physically and mentally.

If limited to a single message, I share the wisdom my wife Diane and I received from a kind, gracious AML survivor:

"Remember, you are a statistic of One."

The survivor referenced the bleak AML mortality statistics but emphasized that each of us is an individual. I accepted the challenge to beat the odds, because I am a statistic of One.

Quality of life is an important aspect of beating cancer. We have a responsibility to ourselves and our loved ones to live life to the fullest. Our days are numbered whether we have cancer or not. Every quality day we have matters and beats cancer.

Please exercise patience with my interspersed, feeble attempts at humor while discussing such a serious subject. But a healthy sense of humor is just as important as a good blood pressure reading.

Finally, I hope to encourage those who face the uncertainty and fear cancer brings.

Diagnosis

December 8, 2020, Prostate surgery. The Mayo Clinic in Rochester, MN was not conducting business as usual. Covid-19 raged across the country, around the world. Hospitals struggled to care for the ever-increasing volume of patients diagnosed with Covid. Political leaders worked on bi-partisan approaches to manage the disease, at least in the beginning.

People delayed doctor visits. Regulators restricted access to medical facilities except for emergencies. Fortunately, the urology department at Mayo remained open for business.

Following a successful robotic surgery, I spent two nights in the hospital and another in a nearby hotel. Diane and I returned home the third day. Recovery required several painless but inconvenient weeks. Mine proceeded as hoped.

The procedure involved removing the prostate, along with over a dozen lymph nodes. Every night for months, afterward, I experienced multiple bathroom calls. The resulting lack of quality sleep left me in a constant state of exhaustion.

But, reassured this was typical, I tried to carry on life as normal. Spring brought the usual lawn-care and landscape projects, and golf. A Florida golf trip with my brothers in May exhausted me. Ninety-degree weather and an unusual amount of exercise made walking up one flight of stairs to our rental condo a chore. The need to sit at length, catching my breath, brought on concerns of heart trouble. Those, I rationalized as exhaustion from my lack of sleep. Besides, I had no history of heart problems.

A summer of outdoor projects and weekly golf outings awaited my return to Minnesota. Trimming our honeysuckle hedge is a two-hour job. But my lack of stamina changed the two-hour task into a four-hour burden, requiring frequent stops to sit and just breathe. A short flight of stairs became difficult to master. Something clearly was not right.

An extensive backyard project, completed in July by a landscaper, added to my summer workload. The summer was hot and dryer than normal. New plants needed water often. The morning of July 20, 2021, I no longer had the strength to hold the hose up for more than a couple of minutes without resting. The time to stop wondering had come. I had to seek help.

Diane drove me to the nearest hospital emergency room. A brief wait, followed by X-rays and a myriad of other tests, produced answers.

Though no history of heart issues or blood clots existed, I feared a heart blockage or stroke caused my lack of energy and labored breathing.

In a mere two hours, the doctors made their initial diagnosis. A pleasant, middle-aged female doctor, not involved in the testing, entered the room. She asked if anyone had given Diane and me the test results. Most likely, this doctor had delivered unpleasant news to patients throughout her career. But her eyes darted around the room. She looked into mine for mere seconds before flitting away again. I sensed she was nervous.

In a kind, but matter-of-fact manner, she reassured us I had no risk of a heart problem or stroke. An instant of relief ended with the news that my bloodwork revealed the presence of acute myeloid leukemia, a rare and extremely serious disease. We questioned the accuracy of the diagnosis. She assured us the blood test for AML did not err, though they required further testing to determine any nuances and specific subtypes of the disease.

Tongue in cheek, I asked about reconsidering a heart problem or stroke. Those conditions yielded significantly better outcomes. A stint placed inside an artery, or a lifelong regimen of blood thinner, seemed much more acceptable options. But, no, we faced a harsh reality. I had cancer, a deadly leukemia.

The doctors admitted me to the hospital.

The following day, Diane and I met the oncologist. He confirmed the initial diagnosis. He insisted I undergo a bone marrow biopsy to help him choose treatment options.

A bone marrow biopsy. The procedure with an awful reputation for those unfamiliar with it. A nurse practitioner or physician assistant drills into the ilium (upper bones making up the hips) to extract the bone marrow samples. The procedure can be painful, including, of course, the possibility of infection.

After a strong recommendation to undergo the biopsy, the doctor sat in silence. He stared into my eyes, a kind but insistent stare. The decision was mine. He had clearly stated that foregoing the procedure limited his ability to choose the optimal course of treatment.

The unfamiliar world of medicine began to open to me. Anxiety always accompanies the unknown. With no time to research the situation, no time to gather my own facts, I had to decide. Everything about this doctor put me at peace. I trusted him and agreed to the procedure.

Extracting the marrow samples took about twenty minutes. A local dose of lidocaine, to numb the area, stung less than a honeybee. In a matter of seconds, the physician assistant proceeded. I experienced no pain. Diane held my hand with daughter-in-law, Cassandra, sitting beside her, supporting us both. Diane squeezed hard, tightening her grip on my hand. But her considerable sense of nervousness and resulting force exerted on my hand hurt more than the damage done by the needles to my back. We all had a laugh.

Lying on my back to prevent bleeding, I rested a few minutes and reflected. These people knew what they were doing... so far. I began to trust my medical team.

Another day passed. Diane and I met again with the oncologist. The biopsy results further categorized the type of AML. The doctor wanted to proceed right away with chemotherapy treatments.

I asked what would happen if I simply went home foregoing the benefit of chemo. Giving me the expected degree of disclaimer, he said I may live three to five days, or three to five weeks or, maybe three to five months.

His response made complete sense to me. My white blood count, the virus fighters, was at 3.5, the extreme, low end of the standard range. My platelets, which cause blood to clot for healing wounds, scored a 38. Anything below 150 was under the normal range. Hemoglobin, red blood cells providing oxygen to the body, scored 6.7. This measure should be above 13. Hence, the lack of energy.

Based on the numbers and the way I felt, surviving three to five weeks might be a stretch.

My doctor recommended two primary courses of action, emphasizing my age and overall good health.

He described the standard treatment as the 'atomic bomb approach.' After enduring a bombardment of high dose, strong chemotherapy for a week, the patient remains under observation, in the hospital, for a month. This effective approach was dangerous for patients over the age of sixty. Devastating side effects often resulted.

He suggested an alternative, referred to as 'the gentler method.' I would be given a new medication, taken at home once each day. In addition, I would receive lower doses of chemo at the clinic for seven days each week. After three weeks, the treatment would be repeated until, with a strong dose of good fortune, I gained remission.

Curing my leukemia was not the objective of either method. The hope was to put the cancer into remission, allowing for a bone marrow transplant. Without a transplant, AML returns within months in nearly every case. But the transplant option did not exist unless we first achieved remission.

The doctor left, leaving us to consider those treatment choices, or the option of doing nothing.

Diane and I stood alone in the room.

I said, "It's a death sentence."

At best, with treatment, I had a 25-30% chance of living beyond five years. I would be seventy-five in five years. Suddenly, that seemed too young. It's more than enough for a lifetime, but when it's personalized, it's too short. My parents died at age seventy-five. Everyone in my family believed seventy-five was too young.

We hugged and cried. This cannot be happening. The bizarre chain of events beginning less than forty-eight hours earlier became increasingly unbelievable. The awful dream continued. A mysterious disease had attacked my blood, and 21st century medical science did not know the cause.

I had no one to blame. Genetics does not tie the disease to parents or family members. Research, thus far, linked no environmental cause to the disease. And apparently neither eating habits nor lack of physical exercise caused AML.

And I did not blame God. Determining what God chooses for us has always been an exercise in frustration and inconclusive guesswork.

Our sons, siblings, and friends needed to hear the news. We made the first calls to our kids. We are a close family. Those calls were gut-wrenching. I did not leave false hope in the form of 'everything will be okay.' A lifelong realist, I taught our boys to expect trouble and hard times. Difficulties would present themselves from time to time. Life is sometimes challenging and painful. And our wealthy western culture, a world focused on material things and the pursuit of a good life, is not immune. I tried to leave them with hope, promising to consider my options with an emphasis on quality of life, not quantity.

Later in the afternoon, my son Brian's family came to the hospital for a visit. Ten and eleven-years-old, at the time, the grandkids were visibly upset. As I stood to greet them, both kids came over crying and hugged me, holding tight for a long minute. Everyone cried.

I'm not sure what I said. Can't remember. The significance of the moment, of embracing those precious little people, overshadowed the need for words.

Family

Sleep that night was anything but restful. The end of life did not affect me as expected. My philosophy is to live every day without expectations for the next. The caveat is to plan for the future while living for the day.

My mind focused on my family. Family. I am the patriarch of the Minnesota clan of my family of origin. My sibling's families, and Diane's, live in North Carolina, Mississippi, Florida, Georgia, and Tennessee. The Minnesota clan consists of our two sons' families, Diane, and me. Our sons, daughters-in-law and four grandchildren live nearby in Minnesota.

Why do I mention them so specifically? Because they mean the world to me. Their troubles are my troubles and their triumphs become mine. I continue to mentor our sons, Brian and Jordan, less like a parent and more like a close friend. They are my best friends. My daughters-in-law and grandchildren are my joy. They are wonderful people who make me tired with their exuberance for and hectic, never-ending pursuit of life. There is little more necessary to say.

Struggling to sleep, thoughts turned to them. My passing would, of course, impact each of them differently. No more mentoring. No more sharing their problems. No more barbeques. No watching them grow or having the kids sit on my lap. No more holidays or vacations to share. No football, soccer games or county fair competitions to watch. No graduations or weddings to attend.

Missing life with my family concerned me more than the thought of dying. It was Thursday night with chemo prep scheduled to begin Friday morning. Sometime late into the night, I decided on another meeting with the doctor before proceeding. Would starting treatments on Monday, instead of Saturday, make any difference? The weekend with my family suddenly became a real priority. This could be the last time I would see them. And I wanted the extra days to consider treatment options.

A nurse brought in medication early Friday, meant as a prep for the following day's start of chemotherapy. I politely refused and asked to meet with the doctor.

As I waited, my daughter-in-law, Cassandra, came by for a visit. An RN with previous experience working on an oncology floor, we relied on her as an excellent resource. She had seen the best and plenty of the worst. I am certain she spared us details, and I respected her effort to protect Diane and me from the reality of possible horrible outcomes. Yet, our visit, after a while, became emotional. She sat next to me on the bedside. Hugging me, we cried.

Diane spent the evening before at home, returning before the doctor arrived.

I was not sure how he would react to my appeal for delaying treatment. But I was aware of one significant risk. Upon first entering the hospital, the emergency room confirmed I tested negative for Covid-19. Contracting the virus over the weekend could delay treatments, not to mention the possibility of serious consequences.

I had no ability to fight infection. The hospital was the safest place. Also, my illness might advance at a rapid pace, rendering any regimen of therapeutics ineffective and hopeless.

An affable fellow, my doctor articulated the difficult subject of life and death with a gentle but plain-spoken approach. Afterward, he listened to our questions. Having a physician willing to listen was extremely gratifying.

A course in the art of empathizing with patients should be required for every upper-level med school curriculum. Upper level so the information is fresh as doctors begin internships. Teaching bedside-manner would be challenging. Personality and life experiences develop a person's ability to step into the shoes of others. Ego has no place in the doctor/patient relationship.

This doctor either aced the course on empathy, or life experiences taught the importance of coming alongside his patients. In each meeting, he penned notes of everything he told us as he explained terms and confirmed our understanding. He handed his scribblings to us for our reference. We felt fortunate this man was on our side. He was well-liked by everyone we encountered in the hospital.

He pointed out that delaying treatments may be a mistake, but probably wasn't. Did he honestly think I had little chance of survival, regardless of which day we started chemo? My mind began to play guessing games, which continued for months to come. I wanted to trust the medical staff. But trusting requires positive experiences and, as I have said, this was new to me. Of course, the decision rested with me. Medical professionals should not make the final decision. But decisions have consequences. And, besides health risks, without the doctor's agreement, checking out of the hospital can create a nightmare with insurance coverage.

After admitting the unusual nature of my appeal, the doctor affirmed his preference for beginning treatment as soon as possible. I promised to keep my distance from anyone with a cold, or worse viruses, and he agreed. I would leave the hospital and return three days later. Granted, the delay presented an element of risk, but a deep-seated fear of not seeing my family again ruled my decision.

Tears came to my eyes during each phone call as we organized our family events for the coming weekend. The possibility this might be my last time with them haunted me. Siblings and cousins offered to fly in from out of state for a visit. Unfortunately, exposure to more people presented too much risk, especially after their close contact with others through travel. Sadly, Diane and I declined their offers.

That weekend, our family shared meals and fished off the docks at the lake. We hugged and cried. The time together will forever remain special to each of us.

On Sunday, the doctor called with additional information from my bone marrow biopsy, and to discuss our final decision concerning treatment.

Until that day, I seriously considered doing nothing. The doctor presented the gentler treatment option as viable. But I had doubts. The gentle approach must be less effective than the preferred primary treatment.

Remission was the best outcome of either approach, and both required a subsequent bone marrow transplant. Questions remained about the transplant. But, at this point, halting the lethal cancer's advance was the goal.

There is wisdom in gathering information. Especially with serious outcomes at stake. But events unfolded faster than we found answers. The situation required a decision.

Family members conferenced in on the doctor's call. I agreed to treatment. We would check into the hospital to begin the gentle chemo approach the next day.

Once settled, tough decisions bring a sense of relief. And though the unknown remains, taking the crucial first step helps with the decisions that follow.

Cancer patients had endured chemotherapy for decades before me. And others before me had tested the gentler chemo protocol. The odds of either treatment did not favor a successful outcome. But with encouragement from my family, we chose to fight AML together, at least for a time.

A Glass Half Full

Enduring the relentless barrage of cancer treatments requires excellent medical providers, unwavering support, dedicated caregivers, and an ever-positive attitude.

An unwillingness to consider the role of attitude can impact the desired outcome. Nothing from my experience is more key to beating AML, or any cancer, than a positive outlook. I believe attitude is at least 80% of facing any challenge.

A controlling personality does not easily rely on the decisions of others. And admittance to a hospital requires just that. I do not have to admit to being a somewhat controlling person. Others have said it for me. There must be some truth to it. Well, okay, there is much truth to it. I'd like to think my controlling persona applies only to the matter of personal safety, but probably not.

For example, my career traveling about the world required frequent plane flights. For the first ten years or so, I approached flying as a necessary but nervous adventure. But my handful of troublesome flights did not help. Lengthy bouts of turbulence or aborted landings to avoid planes on the runway increased my anxiety. Admittedly, I have said I would prefer flying the airplane myself, though I do not know how.

Unsurprisingly, I found surrendering my health care to others a difficult proposition. From my first day in the hospital to start treatments, taking care of myself pretty much ended.

I do not suggest anyone accept every pill and procedure. To advocate for self requires asking questions.

But trust comes into play. Choosing my medical team required a certain amount of trust. And my confidence in their decisions required an attitude adjustment on my part.

But attitude plays another, more important, role. The glass must remain half full. If a glass half empty suggests a negative approach, beating AML requires a glass continually well beyond half full.

My lifelong philosophy has the glass half full, but as stated earlier, I am a realist. Approaching AML with eyes wide open can lead to despair. The statistics of this awful disease are horrible. An unrestrained focus on the numbers can empty the glass to the bottom.

After deciding to fight the cancer, the next step was to ensure I approached each procedure, each day, each setback, in the best frame of mind possible. A simple tool helped.

My son, Brian, and Diane set up an account for me on a website called 'Caring Bridge.' They sent emails and texts to friends and family announcing our plan for using the site to communicate my journey.

Friends and family gained the ability to read our posts with an option to comment. A lifelong fan of football, I adopted the game as an analogy for my fight with cancer. Significant successes and procedures moved the ball closer to the goal line, a complete cure. Setbacks stopped my advance or resulted in negative yardage.

Encouraging responses and 'likes' began to appear on the website. Weekly, I made posts and responded to comments. This quickly became an aid to keeping my spirits high.

As treatments continued through August and September 2021, I encountered cancer patients at various stages of their illness. In the clinic waiting room, some wore scarves covering baldness, others sat in wheelchairs or walked with canes. On each visit, I observed serious difficulties, much more so than those I experienced.

From the beginning, I have said the cancer did not cause me physical pain. Though deadly, my disease had not progressed into discomfort. Neither had my treatments. My problem, so far, was weakness, a complete loss of energy.

Clearly, from what I witnessed at the clinic; others were less fortunate. If I opened the door to depression, even a crack, it seemed a selfish denial of the problems my fellow cancer patients faced.

A proper frame of mind can fend off depression. I am not a psychologist but have lived long enough to witness how the dark place of depression can destroy lives. Depression takes hold like a thief, sneaking in quietly, unnoticed. A deadly disease in its own right, just as cancer cells multiply and divide out of control, depression hitches a ride on weakness and turmoil. Cancer creates not only physical but also mental frailty and trouble.

Doctors, physician assistants, nurse practitioners, registered nurses, nurse's assistants, dieticians, supply people and hospital cleaning staff are human beings. Each person has life struggles.

I became somewhat acquainted with medical personnel during my clinic visits and long days in the hospital. During each visit, different nurses administered my treatments. We interacted like co-workers on a passenger airplane, crews meeting for a single flight before going our separate ways for the next.

As they treated my cancer, we shared conversations. It's amazing how personal problems come to light between people mildly acquainted. Who knows what made them comfortable sharing with me? Maybe my willingness to listen or maybe they found an old guy easy to talk to. Regardless, opportunities arose to encourage them in their work, their dreams and sometimes their problems. Encouraging others has always had a positive impact on my personal state of mind.

My medical team and caregivers have commented time and again on my positive attitude. It takes work, at times, but has remained as much a part of my cure as the chemo, radiation, and medical know how.

Side Effects

No one is immune to the constant barrage of televised drug advertisements. Marketing pitches spend as much time making disclaimers and discussing potential side effects as they do on the medicine's effectiveness.

Side effects. Those with any exposure to cancer treatments are aware of the myriad of possible reactions. They range from discomfort to painful and debilitating. The adage is: 'doctors attempt to kill the cancer without killing the patient.'

But where there is bad news, something positive can be found. One result of treatment is weight loss. Doctors and dieticians advised us that chemo treatments and the stem cell transplant might cause me to lose up to fifteen pounds. For me, this was welcome news.

Two years before discovering my prostate cancer, I began a serious effort to lose weight. By the time AML treatments began, my successful effort left me fifteen pounds short of my goal. Dropping more excess pounds would be welcomed, but I feared losing too much. I adopted the 'eat anything you want diet.' Milkshakes, a high calorie treat I denied myself the past thirty years, became a staple. Orange juice, normally avoided, was no longer a concern.

Birthday cakes. A few years before the cancers, I developed a strong appreciation for a particular style cake made at the bakery of a local grocery store. The icing is thick and wonderful. I like a little cake with my icing. And having the bakery add a lengthy name required another scrumptious layer of pure sugary icing.

Whenever the craving hit me, I rationalized that someone, somewhere, celebrated a birthday. In February, for example, I would have my impromptu cake decorated atop the already thick icing with 'Happy Birthday, Abraham Lincoln.'

Birthday cake became a staple for my 'eat anything you want' diet. The lifelong battle to watch calories ended, temporarily.

Thank goodness medical advances have reduced the negative effects of cancer therapies. Yet, multiple common chemotherapy side effects remain. And these can occur any time throughout treatment and years afterward.

A plethora of drugs exist to minimize cancer treatment side effects. But patients do not recognize some negative effects, such as the impact of chemo on the kidneys or liver. Organs are monitored and additional meds administered to protect them from the chemo. It's a mind blowing, endless stream of oral and intravenous drugs. Drugs, drugs, and more drugs.

My experience with adverse effects may have been atypical. I had no major reactions during weeks of chemotherapy. No nausea, vomiting, diarrhea, skin rash, headaches, or seizures.

Early on, though, I had an episode of chemo-brain. Also known as chemo-fog, cognitive impairment occurs affecting concentration and causing difficulty with speech. Tasks take longer to complete, and a general feeling of fogginess sets in, all of which can be frustrating.

Family members noticed my inability to choose words during a conversation. I was tongue-tied at times. Typing became more challenging. Not impossible, but difficult. I considered quitting until the condition improved.

The chemo-brain did not significantly impair my ability to communicate. And the effects lasted no more than a couple of weeks, causing minimal frustration.

Weeks after chemo treatments began, a mouth sore developed behind my molars, painful to the degree that swallowing became difficult. A diet of soft food helped, but my body had no ability to heal the sore. Chemo drugs, as planned, had killed my white blood cells. A lack of those virus fighting cells left me vulnerable, unable to heal a simple mouth sore.

Eating mushy food for a few days can result in the loss of several pounds. So, this is what the doctors meant by weight loss. The only food or liquid possible to swallow, with acceptable pain, on my 'eat anything you want' diet, was milkshakes. But those, too, caused significant discomfort.

Magic Mouthwash. A physician assistant at the clinic prescribed a concoction referred to as Magic Mouthwash. The plan was to swish this solution throughout my mouth multiple times each day. While easing the pain right away, the sore would slowly cure. It didn't do either.

In a chance conversation with a different physician assistant, she suggested a more effective prescription solution. After swishing the new liquid for several days, the pain stopped, and the ulcer disappeared. I have renamed the concoction Miracle Mouthwash.

I learned two important aspects of advocacy from this episode. First, keep asking until every possibility is exhausted. Second, no medical expert has all the answers. Experience matters. And their experiences are as diverse as their education and the places they have worked. Present the question to different providers if the first doesn't resolve the issue.

Though troubling and painful, I considered the mouth ulcer a minor side effect. An extended battle with mouth and throat sores, and the resulting diet of mushy and liquid foods, can cause excessive weight loss. But my episode, fortunately, lasted less than a week.

Weeks passed and a more agonizing side effect surfaced, constipation. Many have experienced this from time to time, but not me. To avoid discussing the indelicate particulars, let's just say constipation can be a horrible result of chemotherapy.

Once again, my interest in food subsided. My system had no room. Any number of cures exist, but this condition worsens by the hour to become excruciating. You might say the problem snuck up on me from behind.

Normal treatments offered no relief. Increasing dosages of over-the-counter methods did not help. In the 'end,' large doses of MiraLAX proved successful. The relief is indescribable. I insisted that constipation is worse than cancer.

Another bout with obstructed guts occurred the next week. This was every bit as uncomfortable. But an early dose of MiraLAX resolved my dilemma. I became a quick learner.

Each treatment cycle, nurses gave me two painless cancer shots for seven consecutive days in the clinic. One day, I mentioned my recurring constipation problem to a nurse. She admitted a nausea prevention drug, given before the shots, often caused constipation. She further indicated I may not need the medication. I figured nausea could not be as bad as my horrible cases of constipation. Anything was worth a try.

I declined the anti-nausea med. The result, no more constipation and no nausea. A chance conversation with the right nurse solved the problem. This, again, reinforced the need to advocate for myself and ask questions of different medical providers.

Sixty days after therapy began, my doctor ordered another bone marrow biopsy. To the delight of everyone, the treatments achieved complete remission in a mere two months. We had moved the football to the thirty-yard line, first down and ten. The clock ticked toward the next step, a stem cell transplant.

Chemotherapy continued with the goal of keeping me in remission.

We scheduled a consultation with the University of Minnesota transplant team for mid-October. That consult never happened.

At a weekly clinic appointment in October, I reported pain in my right side. A particularly clever physician assistant recommended a CT scan.

We went to an affiliated clinic near our home for the scan. Afterward, I returned home and went to bed. I continued to feel worse. The pain grew more intense by the hour. My fever had increased but not yet reached the 100.5 °F benchmark, triggering an immediate trip to the emergency room.

Not long after lying down, Diane came in with a message from the doctor's office. The CT scan confirmed the pain in my side, appendicitis. I literally laughed out loud. Prostate cancer in 2020, AML in 2021, and now, appendicitis. The discovery of a new, dangerous malady wasn't funny. Rather, it struck me as so ridiculous, I had to laugh. My offensive movement stopped well short of the goal line, dead in its tracks. This setback left me at fourth and long. An unexpected attacker had sacked my quarterback.

Once again, a quick visit to the hospital ER led to admittance. Further tests over the next couple of days confirmed either appendicitis or a serious infection surrounding my appendix. Not 100% sure, surgeons preferred not to operate. The chemo, as expected, had depleted my blood platelets. An operation could cause excessive bleeding to the point of, potentially, death.

Instead, doctors prescribed a regimen of antibiotics, hoping my low white blood count had caused an infection. The plan worked. The infection surrounding my appendix was, without question, a negative effect of the chemo, not appendicitis.

My oncologist suspended the cancer therapy for at least a week, starting again once I recovered.

Treatments continued throughout the balance of October and into November. In late November, blood tests continued to reveal dangerously low levels of white blood cells. My white cells, driven to near extinction by intent, did not bounce back as expected. The inability to fight infection concerned my medical team.

Again, my oncologist paused treatments. This therapy stuff became a moving target. My offense played against a defense that kept changing their formations. This life and death game required my team to make continual adjustments.

I would limp through December, until late January, without chemo. Hopefully, the cancer would remain in remission. A third biopsy, in January, would determine my eligibility for the transplant.

We rescheduled the BMT team consult for late November.

Throughout my treatment, blood count results often dictated infusions of platelets and red blood cells. These, too, are painless side effects of the cancer meds, although infusions come with risks.

The number and severity of treatment side effects for me was low. Some say I downplayed them. But my medical staff agreed my experience was better than many others.

Some patients have existing health issues that contribute to side effects. But otherwise healthy people can react differently. This is a mystery. The medical community admits there is much to learn.

The advice given by the AML survivor to Diane and me comes to mind.

'Remember, you are a statistic of One.'

This applies to side effects too.

Prep Week

Bone marrow transplant is an outdated term. The medical profession is changing the name to 'Stem Cell Transplant.' Stem cells are baby blood cells, those from which other blood cells mature. Bone marrow manufactures stem cells to produce mature blood cells.

Medical professionals would harvest healthy stem cells from an unrelated donor for the type of transplant I needed.

Be The Match. Patients can sometimes use stem cells from family members or their own. But often the search extends to unrelated donors. *Be The Match*, an organization matching donors to recipients, is worldwide in scope. I learned an amazing donor fact from a nurse who attended my full-body radiation. He said the university's transplants are oft times from donors in Germany and Belgium. In fact, *Be The Match* has over 41 million individuals worldwide willing to offer their cells. Doctors prefer donors in the age range of 18-40.

As my oncologist put it, "Stem cells of people over 40 have had too many birthdays."

Donating stem cells is a non-surgical procedure. The miracle of donating organs and stem cells is a phenomenon difficult to appreciate until you know the recipient. Or until you are the recipient. I will forever encourage people to consider becoming a donor.

A BMT nurse searched the *Be The Match* database. She found three donors with specific blood cell markers matching mine at a minimum of 80%. Follow-up identified two individuals available and willing to participate immediately.

My son Jordan's family visited from out of town for the Christmas holiday. As expected, we each had our concerns about my upcoming transplant. And though doctors insisted the procedure itself was not dangerous, the short-term effects could have a deadly outcome.

As Jordan's family left that December, everyone wished me the best. But as they went out the front door, my granddaughter lingered. Seventeen at the time, she stood with me in the kitchen. After an extended hug, she pulled away, looking me in the eye.

"You got this, Grandpa," she said.

I had to look away. A caring teenager gave me a directive, an order of confidence. Her reassurance bolstered my confidence. She usually called me Gramps. But the moment called for the more serious version, Grandpa. Encouragement came from everywhere.

January 13, forty-ninth wedding anniversary. To celebrate, Diane and I toured the University of Minnesota hospital radiation unit. Very interesting, but not quite as exciting as our special day forty-nine years earlier.

January 28, check-in to the hospital.

My room on the Bone Marrow Transplant floor, at Fairview, University of Minnesota Hospital, overlooked the south part of downtown Minneapolis. Below the hill outside my window, the Mississippi River snaked its way through the city, hidden beneath ice and snow.

The view was impressive, though the circumstances lacked any appeal. That isn't completely accurate. Although I would rather be some other place, I was glad the final step in my treatment would happen soon. The last few yards are the toughest close to the goal line.

The expansive room afforded ample space for a massive smart bed, recliner, and cushioned seating area along the windows. The bed could calculate my weight. It also had an alarm system to alert staff for patients with risk of falling.

A table, large enough for a laptop or food tray, stood in the corner with a chair. After meeting with a physical therapist, staff wheeled in a massive stationary peddling machine.

This room was typical in the BMT unit, except for the view. During my stay, nurses disclosed that patients highly sought the room. Some, who returned, requested it. I had no intention of returning. My home for the next thirty days was nice, but my goal was a one and done. Score a touchdown, go home, and stay home.

Several medical tests confirmed the donor's health was acceptable to proceed. With that assurance, I began a weeklong battery of exams. CT scans, EKGs, EEGs, pulmonary tests, and x-rays checked for existing conditions which might disqualify me as a viable candidate.

One test was for Covid. A positive result might not prevent the BMT procedure but could cause unwanted delay. I lost count of the number of Covid tests I endured since my initial visit to Mayo in 2020.

With acceptable test results from the donor and me, a final bone marrow biopsy would determine the status of my cancer. Only then could the medical staff ask the donor to proceed.

My final biopsy confirmed I had remained in remission. To my pleasant surprise, none of the biopsies caused significant pain. My oncologist set the transplant date, Feb. 4, 2022. Now the hard work began. Prep the week before transplant required three days of heavy chemo followed by full body radiation. The radiation is a twenty-minute, painless process.

Once more, the chemicals did their job without causing any noticeable side effects. At times, I wondered about the chemotherapy's effectiveness. If the treatments did not make me nauseous or cause other problems, were they working?

Doctors, PAs, and nurses came and went. A physical therapist dropped in explaining her role. One day, the staff dietician came by for a visit.

When I mentioned the expectation of losing fifteen pounds, she said, "We are not going to let that happen."

I responded, "That doesn't make me very happy."

My reaction surprised her. She elaborated, informing me the staff would use intravenous feeding for patients who did not take in enough calories.

Since my diagnosis earlier in July, my research and comments from medical professionals indicated the transplant process caused significant weight loss. As a result, I not only stopped dieting, I gained back pounds I had worked hard to lose. Making no further comment to the dietician, I resolved to take management of the food issue into my own hands. My goal was to lose at least fifteen pounds.

Prep week ended on a Thursday. Using my football analogy, my team had moved the ball to the ten-yard-line.

Transplant

February 4, 2022, stem cell transplant. Two registered nurses brought three tiny IV pouches into my room. They checked the number code, identifying the bag's contents, double-checking every detail with each other, while confirming a final time, my name and birthdate.

I looked at Diane. Though reassured the induction process had minimal risk, we found ourselves at the point of no return. A new blood-type and new DNA would change my body forever. I relaxed and held one of the pouches. Thick crimson liquid filled the bag, no larger than my hand, with new life. With me sitting in the recliner and holding the first sac of cells, we took a picture and proceeded.

I watched with understandable anticipation as the nurse hung the bag on the IV tower infusion hook, high above the chair. What might my blood pressure reading look like now? As the first red droplet slid into the tubing, the nurse opened the roller clamp, allowing the new cells to march toward my port. Live cells, healthy cells, someone else's cells. Would this really work? Closing my eyes, I attempted to feel the thick new cells enter my veins. Nothing, neither cold nor hot, no pressure. Nothing. Everyone in the room waited in silence.

The next thirty to one-hundred days were critical. And I could have a serious, even deadly, setback for the next two years.

Twenty minutes passed. The last of the three bags hung empty on the IV tower. My stem cell transplant was complete. The protocol required no further procedures for the next twenty-four hours.

Afterward, my medical team infused a regimen of strong chemo for two days. Recent research showed this new procedure could prevent the new cells from attacking and damaging my organs. Next, IVs of saline flushed the meds from my body for twelve hours.

Those were two days of hell. Over those forty-eight hours, I reaffirmed to myself, again and again, a principle I developed long before in life.

'I can handle most anything for a short time.'

Every possible side effect hit me. Well, not all of them. But the results made up for my ability to breeze through the previous five months.

Besides throwing up, uncontrollable diarrhea, loss of appetite, etc., etc., this treatment sapped my energy, which did not return for another three months.

The energy loss is difficult to explain. But a trip across the hospital room to the bathroom on the other side required every ounce of energy I could muster. The short walk resulted in several minutes of heavy breathing. My body experienced a weakness, fatigue unlike anything imaginable.

I mentioned uncontrollable diarrhea, a subject better left in the dark. But a story of my experience must be told.

A physician assistant checked on me after I had struggled with the problem for a full day. At the time, my daughter-in-law, Cassandra, visited with our ten- and eleven-year-old grandkids. Any discussion pertaining to bodily functions is of the utmost interest to people their age. Before answering the PA's questions, I stole a quick glance at the kids. They sat on the edge of their seats, waiting to overhear the foul discussion.

Turning back to the PA, I said, "Well, it has become about the consistency of cream of mushroom soup."

Another glance revealed both grandkids using every ounce of their adolescent control to maintain their composure. With the visit concluded, the PA left, along with my visitors. I grabbed my cell phone and sent a text to my granddaughter, the eleven-year-old who had walked away snickering about my bathroom related dilemma. I knew she had recently completed canning a bunch of pickles.

My text read, "Hey, don't you have some jars leftover from your canning project we could use for the cream of mushroom soup?"

Obviously, I could not see her face, but the response came with plenty of laughing emojis. We have laughed about the incident since, and I suppose we will tell the story for years to come.

The University of Minnesota BMT unit required patients to remain in the hospital for a full month of observation following transplant. This protocol varies among different hospitals.

After recovering from the harsh chemo, the days became long, consisting of as much exercise as possible to prevent pneumonia while regaining my strength.

Doctors placed no food restrictions on me. But hospital food went from borderline okay to borderline disgusting. In fairness, little of anything tasted good. My doctor assured me my sense of taste would improve over the coming months. Visits from Diane and my sons brought burritos and subs from local fast-food restaurants. Finding food acceptable to my palate became a daily chore.

A nurse assistant checked my weight daily. I began to drop pounds. For the first time since my childhood, I appreciated my excess weight. Losing too much became a concern. I forced myself to eat. Eating and exercising required unfailing discipline, a trait I had mastered sporadically throughout life.

The effects of the treatment played mental gymnastics with me. A lifelong mindset of watching my weight ended, temporarily, in no more time than the transplant required.

Though I have a significant sweet tooth, many foods tasted too sweet. Small amounts of sweetener cooked into vegetables, sauces, and breads ruined their taste. Strangely, or not, cake, cookies, ice cream, and candy tasted fine. Also, I found meat of any kind, and pasta, curiously acceptable. Mac and cheese became a staple.

Salad dressings, pizza sauces, fried food, and eggs tasted awful. Fried food. I no longer liked fried food. When I grew up in the south, my mom fried everything but the iced tea. Now, my taste buds shunned one of my favorite foods.

None of this resulted from my new stem cells. Post-transplant required a plethora of meds designed to fight viruses, fungus, respiratory issues, and rejection of the new cells. Certain drugs protected me from certain others. Something in this combination of drugs wreaked havoc with my tastebuds.

Every day, a number of hospital staff members visited. Nursing assistants for checking vitals, freshening my water, changing bedding, and verifying changes in my weight. Physician assistants and nurse practitioners for mini-exams to report back to the docs. Dieticians and physical therapists dropped in from time to time. Cleaning people came daily along with supply staff to refill items used from a cabinet. Mornings resembled rush hour at Grand Central Station. Afternoons quieted down a good bit.

Two doctors from the BMT team visited daily, and a third dropped in weekly. An older doc came with a Fellow, a doctor in his late 30s preparing to specialize in BMT. I became well acquainted with those gentlemen as I did with my nurses, PAs and NPs.

Before I went into the hospital, my older brother sent me the entire set of DVDs for the *Game of Thrones* series. Both of my daily visiting doctors had seen the series and guaranteed I, too, would enjoy it.

My laptop had no DVD player, but surprisingly, my room TV did. But after several attempts, I couldn't get the player to work.

My doctors began to ask how I was enjoying the series. I explained that the DVD player did not work. Both doctors tried their technical expertise. After neither succeeded, the older fellow promised to tell someone at the nurse's station. In five minutes, literally five minutes, a twenty-something registered nurse came into the room. Seconds later, the player functioned perfectly.

The next day, I told the older doctor how the young nurse solved the DVD problem. A few days later, leaving my room, he informed the younger doctor. While shaking his head from side to side, he spoke with a defeatist tone, admitting our reliance upon the younger generation to fix the video player. I smiled. The episode was a highlight of my hospital stay.

A week after my transplant, I noticed hair from my head and beard shedding. It fell out in bunches. Grabbing a handful of beard, and pulling ever so lightly, removed chunks of gray. Now age 71, I had kept, at least, a mustache dating back to college. In recent years, I sported a full, short beard.

I took and sent a selfie to my Minnesota family and my siblings in the south. In the accompanying note, I stated the picture might be invaluable as I prepared to shave my head and beard. Unsurprisingly, I received no agreement on the picture's potential value.

After shaving my beard, mustache and hair, the result resembled the actor, Bruce Willis, from his famous movie, *Die Hard*. Screwing my face into a sullen scowl, I took another selfie. The reactions provided plenty of laughter. The BMT experience is, frankly, not much fun. Providing a bit of levity, whenever the opportunity arose, was helpful to my family as well as me.

Aside from the two days of chemo after the transplant, little changed in the days that followed. My strength showed marginal improvement, though I exercised daily. The BMT patient rooms form a triangle surrounding the nursing station. Each trip through the hallways measures 1/10th of a mile. I began with 3 trips and increased my walks to 10 over a matter of days. Those short strolls exhausted me.

One day, while walking the halls, I passed a male nurse. Identifying me as a patient by the stainless-steel IV tree I pushed along, he stopped me.

He said, "The quickest way out of here is little circles around these halls."

That short moment of encouragement was one of many helping to keep my glass half-full.

Going home required my blood counts to hit certain benchmarks. My white blood count did not cooperate, a recurring theme since cancer treatments started in August.

Week four in the hospital, I received a med designed as a white blood cell growth factor. A similar drug worked wonders the previous October. Within twenty-four hours, tests showed my counts began to recover. After another forty-eight hours, my white blood cells returned to the normal range.

Isolation

Thursday, February 24, going home a full week earlier than scheduled. My blood count numbers for every measure hit acceptable ranges the day before, and I guess the docs and nurses were ready to get rid of me.

But seriously, considering the many nurses attending me day in and day out, only one behaved curt and hurried. I gave her the benefit of the doubt. Everyone has those days. And a nurse's job is constant stop and start, running from one patient to another. They steal bits of time for food and bathroom breaks, often entering a patient's room to face the unexpected.

Discharge: The nurse on duty outfitted me with a shopping bag full of meds. Antiviral, antifungal, anti-pneumonia, anti-rejection, and anti-GVHD, along with others designed to decrease potential side effects from the anti-meds. Topping off the hefty bag were my standard blood pressure and cholesterol pills, old buddies I had taken for years. The bag included a sizeable pill box and an assortment of printed sheets, instructions for the meds.

Another nurse dropped by to give us a short course on home care for my Hickman catheter. A surgeon installed the device in my chest during my prep week. Used for implanting the stem cells, the port remained in place until May for follow up blood work.

Along the hallway, past the nurse's station, Diane and I stopped to thank those on duty. Using my knuckle, a Covid habit, I pushed the elevator button. A bustle of people milled about the main floor. They filled the chairs lining the hospital entrance waiting room. I wanted everyone to know I had survived. Of course, none of them knew what I had been through. Every person chatting or on their phones, sat waiting for someone else.

Automatic doors opened as we approached the front entrance. I breathed the first fresh air in weeks. My immature immune system required me to wear a mask outdoors for the next seventy days. Regardless, freedom from the hospital environment came with a sense of excitement. Don't get me wrong, my hospital experience, though confining, wasn't terrible. But it wasn't home.

One of our living room chairs occupies a spot at the corner of the sofa, beside a wide picture window. It's 'my chair,' the one I sit in every day, working on my novels. Twenty feet above the backyard, the window offers a full view of acres of magnificent marshland. Our bird feeder, my daytime distraction, hangs just outside the window. I made straight for the chair. The distance from our garage to 'my chair' is a mere fifteen steps, but the short walk exhausted me.

For the first few minutes, I sat reflecting on the previous two months. I was not the same person. An abundance of medical professionals changed me, saving me from myself, from my self-destructing blood cells.

My surreal journey continued. I suppose anyone who encounters any form of cancer can relate. Nothing about it seemed real. There I sat, in the comfort of my home, still alive, still here for my family.

Empty for weeks, the bird feeder swung in a slight breeze, devoid of activity. Feeding the birds was my job, but I had busied myself with other things. The marsh scene changed little since I left in January. Clumps of reed grasses struggled to reveal themselves from late February snow cover.

Winter can produce weeks of gray, but the sky this day displayed a deep, bright blue, as if a thunderstorm had cleared the air. Like a medical thunderstorm had cleared my bone marrow of defective blood cells.

Covid-19 somewhat prepared us for BMT isolation. By late 2021, everyone had experienced degrees of detachment from each other, an eerie disruption of normal human interaction. Long distance travel became difficult and rare. Masks created a hemmed-in feeling during routine shopping visits. Shaking hands ended. And 'smiling' with the eyes required practice, a skill worth the extra effort for passing people in the store.

My hundred days from transplant would not end until mid-May. The confinement was like Covid-19 isolation on steroids. My doctor insisted I have a caregiver available 24/7. I could only stay alone for an hour at most. Reminiscent of when our kids were small, we put together a list of sitters, those willing to sit with me, allowing Diane to run errands or take a break for herself.

Friends and family filled the void. Those still working brought their laptops. I sat in my chair working on a book while visiting with my sitters. Those visits did not seem necessary, but each one was special.

My medical team had warned us a serious episode of GVHD could occur quickly.

I had the good fortune of experiencing no incident of any kind while visitors stayed with me in our home. On one occasion, a neighbor sat for a while. His wife came by later to relieve him for a meeting he had scheduled. Jokingly, I asked if he told her what to do should I pass out.

Without missing a beat, he said to her, "Go through his wallet and take his credit cards."

Isolation meant more than just staying at home. An immature immune system requires an extensive list of restrictions. Avoiding dust and mold was paramount. As mentioned before, if I stepped outside, I needed a mask. Diane dusting or vacuuming required me to leave the room. Moldy foods, such as blue cheese dressing, were dangerous. Of course, blue cheese is my favorite, by far. As Covid restrictions slowed, salad and hot food bars opened again at local restaurants and grocery stores. Those remained off limits, compliments of my compromised immune system.

We ordered meals for delivery and picked up consumable items. We took advantage of new services allowing pickup at stores. Of course, Amazon came in handy. Friends and family dropped off items at the front door. My infrequent outings consisted of accompanying Diane to the store and waiting in the car while she shopped.

The rules of my recovery protocol did not allow me to drive. A reaction to my meds or the mysterious, debilitating, GVHD attack might occur. Fortunately, it never did.

Nothing had restricted my ability to drive since I got my license as a teenager. No injury to my ankles or legs or long-term illness had robbed me of my ability to go where I wanted whenever I wanted. Isolation provided a glimpse of the freedom we lose later in life after age takes away the privilege of driving.

My medical team allowed us to entertain visitors, two or three at once, but absolutely no one with an illness or Covid symptoms. Kids and grandkids dropped by for short visits, sitting across the room or standing outside the front door.

My uninspired appetite lingered, affecting my calorie intake. At least twice each week, a chocolate milkshake supplemented my otherwise meager diet. I avoided my favorite pizza from a local restaurant. My sense of taste had become so limited, I feared ruining forever my enjoyment of what I claim is the best pizza in Minnesota. Weight loss continued.

I understood how important isolation was and fully embraced it. Isolation was a means to an end. I knew that years later, this entire bizarre ordeal would seem like just a moment in time. My days sheltering away now could help me make it to that future time.

In March, a significant rash appeared on my neck, chest, and shoulders, GVHD. My new blood cells had attacked my skin. An exam by an astute Physician Assistant resulted in a prescription for two creams. One for my face and neck and a second, more aggressive, for my chest.

Her comment was, "We have to teach the new cells your skin is not a threat, and they will settle down."

Three times each day Diane helped apply the creams. Within the week, any evidence of a rash disappeared. Unfortunately, the episode affected the schedule for tapering off my anti-rejection medication. I had to take the drug two weeks longer, into August. But if this was the worst effect of Guest Versus Host Disease, the short extension was acceptable.

Every incident, such as the rash, or a slight fever, or uneasy stomach, brought a hint of fear. Any of those could be serious, an indication my new stem cells were working against me.

But dwelling on the negative changes nothing. I accepted the new normal for my health. And though

I'm not a particularly introspective person, from now on, I needed to pay attention to signals from my body.

Each day, we moved one day closer to the end. Each week, one week closer. And though we counted the days, I cannot say my quarantine was a total drudge. Isolation provided plenty of time for writing. I finished the third novel in my series based on the lives of Mary Queen of Scots and her son, King James I.

I continued the exercises sent home by physical therapy. My energy slowly increased. But my appetite remained poor.

Beyond 100 Days

Isolation ended May 17, one-hundred, and two days after my transplant. A bone marrow biopsy on May 11, and resulting consultations, pushed the hundred days out a couple. We welcomed more excellent news from the biopsy. My bone marrow continued to contain 100% donor cells. No hint of leukemia.

A lesser regimen of medications continued. My doctor scheduled the anti-rejection medication, Tacrolimus, to phase out over the summer. I continued treatments of Pentamidine every month, a med inhaled to prevent pneumonia.

And my old standby, the anti-viral Acyclovir, continued as well. I began taking Acyclovir with my initial chemotherapy in July 2021. In the spring of 2023, the need for this med ended, the last of innumerable drugs taken over almost two years.

My oncologist stressed the importance of avoiding dust and mold. She emphasized my immature immune system. This meant a summer without yardwork or fishing. A restriction against any major home projects continued as well.

Diane and I decided to take a road trip soon after isolation ended. My doctor approved as long as we followed existing Covid precautions and avoided visiting anyone with illness.

June 11, Diane and I set out on a driving trip from Minnesota to Mississippi, Georgia, and North Carolina, returning after eleven days. We visited twenty-two relatives and drove through thirteen states. I played four rounds of golf, my first since fall.

My first round was on top of Lookout Mountain, Georgia, with my brother-in-law. The temperature soared to a sultry 95°F. At one-hundred and twenty days after transplant, admittedly, my energy had not yet returned to 100%. To make matters worse, I dressed in long sleeves and pants to avoid the sun.

The golf was enjoyable, but the weather, nearly unbearable. My brother-in-law wore shorts and short sleeves, which offered him little comfort. Needless to say, I survived. I learned that slathering on 70spf suntan lotion to wear shorts was much better than long pants and sleeves.

The next three rounds of golf, the weather and my scores improved. But I did not score better than before my transplant. I told everyone I wanted stem cells from a lady who was an excellent golfer. I figured the combination might make me better looking and improve my golf scores. No offense to my male donor, but neither has happened.

No one we visited had Covid, but the week after our return, Diane and I noticed symptoms. A quick check confirmed the virus. Concerned my immune system might not provide adequate protection, I was fortunate to only experience a slight loss of energy and cold symptoms.

Summer passed in a hurry. I continued to avoid dirt, mold, and dust. But the first week in September, a mystery illness put me in the hospital.

I had scheduled a round of golf with my son, Brian, but felt poorly the day before the outing. My desire to visit with my son and play a popular course motivated me to try. After struggling through the first nine holes, I decided to ride along in the cart the last nine.

The next morning, my temperature hit 100.8°F, exceeding the threshold for a trip to the emergency room. BMT staff directed me to a local clinic for a quick Covid test. To my surprise, I tested positive.

At the hospital, aides whisked us away to a room isolating Covid patients. Any medical personnel entering my room donned special suits for their protection. They began blood tests to determine the cause of my fever and soon shuttled me to a room on the BMT unit, again isolated from other patients.

Shortly, a Physician Assistant I recognized came in to visit. She wore no protective Covid gear.

I asked, "Where's your space suit?"

Through her traditional face mask, she said, "Oh, you don't have Covid."

By this time, I had learned that nothing related to medicine would surprise me.

The PA continued, "They run the test through a number of iterations to determine if the virus is present. Yours showed up on one of the last iterations. You only have a residual amount of Covid from your bout with it last June. You're not contagious."

Her explanation made sense. Why other medical staff members dressed in 'space suits' and plastic face shields made no sense.

Initial blood tests indicated my white blood count had dropped to almost zero. I had no neutrophils, those tiny white blood cells whose job is to fight infections of any kind. After a couple of days waiting for lab results, the staff diagnosed an infection in my intestines, the probable result of my immature immune system. Apparently, an infection had wiped out my white blood cells.

They did not know why or how to proceed. And these people are extremely capable in their area of expertise. The medical team actually voted on a course of treatment.

I needled my doctor, "I was okay until I found out you guys voted on how to solve my problem."

She responded, "Honestly, we are guessing. This is beyond science."

The best medical minds in the world of bone marrow transplants just admitted they questioned the treatment options. My good friend from college told me a simple truth forty years before, in the early years of his surgery practice. He said there is so much we don't know.

Most people intuitively understand that, but with your personal health in question, the reality that doctors don't know everything about every illness can be difficult to accept.

A regimen of antibiotics and prednisone began. The medical team's vote concerned the dosage and duration of prednisone treatment, a drug best taken for short periods.

I received a minor dose in the hospital, and a prescription phased out over the coming weeks. The steak and glass of bourbon I planned for my upcoming golf trip to TPC Sawgrass became a steak, and virgin Marguerita. Admittedly a trifling sacrifice. Nevertheless, sacrifices had become the norm. At least I was not prohibited from going.

The plan worked.

In the short-term, this episode resulted in nothing more than an empty bourbon glass. But for the long-term it threatened to affect my glass half full attitude. I will forever be wary of the onset of GVHD. The effects, as stated earlier, can be devastating, including the possibility of death.

After the September hospital stay, October through the next January passed without incident. I began to gain weight. By the time of my first BMT anniversary, February 2023, I had gained back the pounds lost, plus another ten.

I commented to Diane, "I am completely off my 'Eat anything you want' diet. The need to manage my weight gives me a good feeling. It's an indication I'm alive."

Caregivers

A cancer diagnosis is an attack on the whole person. Emotions run unrestrained, from horror to dread to hope, and even to peace. Families and friends struggle with acceptance.

After the initial shock, everyone follows the victim through months and sometimes years of treatments to cure or death. This is especially true for the Caregiver.

A Caregiver's duties differ depending upon the particular illness. On a scale of 1 to 10, with 10 the most difficult, caring for an AML patient who has had a stem cell transplant is probably a 9.

For transplant patients, the Caregiver must be available 24hours/day for weeks and months. Their responsibilities become more intensive and time consuming, bordering on the unbearable, after the patient receives a stem cell transplant.

In most cases, the Caregiver is a relative, someone willing to sacrifice their time, rearranging their life on the patient's behalf. My Caregiver is my wife, Diane. We have been married fifty years.

As mentioned earlier, the BMT team at the University of Minnesota Hospital performed my transplant. Their protocol required a thirty-day hospital stay.

February in Minnesota can be an excellent month to stay indoors. Unless you are a regular winter sports participant. The timing for a transplant in February sounded good to us.

But this can be a challenging month on the roads. We live twenty minutes from the hospital and clinic. The route is interstate from the suburbs to downtown. Diane made trip after trip, too often in ice and snow. She drove frequently in heavy traffic. After my return home in March, we visited the clinic, day after day, week after week, for checkups to include an occasional infusion of red blood cells or platelets. Minnesota weather in March is marginally better than February for driving on crowded interstates.

Each day, during the seventy days of isolation, Diane helped flush my Hickman port with saline solution. This became routine. But it can be intimidating for people not trained in medical procedures. Especially if a loved one is involved.

Some patients return to the clinic daily to have professionals care for their ports. Everyone's comfort level is different. We preferred managing the awkward, but simple, port flush at home. That option suited us better than climbing into the car to navigate traffic and weather for more clinic visits.

Caregivers must take charge of the patient's eating habits. I had no interest in food and most of it did not taste normal. My doctor said to eat anything, consume as many calories as possible. She emphasized volume over quality, calories over taste.

My Caregiver experienced days of frustration in her constant attempt to feed me.

Diane needed to leave the house for shopping, errands, or a bit of free time. This required an extensive effort to schedule visitors willing to sit with me. While at home, she remained dedicated to the task, a full-time job of caring and giving.

I have mentioned a few occasions which emphasized, to me, the importance of advocating for myself. To achieve the best results in anything requires gathering as much information as possible. This applies to medical issues as well. Never assume. Ask questions and be comfortable with disagreeing. It's every person's right.

But a patient's condition can affect their memory or render them unable to think clearly. Caregivers and others, available as often as possible, can help. An extra set of eyes and ears to communicate with medical providers is invaluable.

Diane was ever busy with food prep, shopping, house cleaning, scheduling, driving, applying medicated lotion, flushing my port, listening in, and recording calls with doctors, and clinic visits. She supported me during medical procedures, and simply visiting. Caregivers set aside their own life temporarily.

Do not take a Caregiver for granted. They perform this selfless task under emotional and physical stress. They are generous, caring, people. Special people.

I am forever grateful for Diane's sacrifice.

No One Gets a Trophy

Victory: The result of winning a battle, success against a foe.

The medical community has come far in its war against cancer. Researchers have worked for hundreds of years to understand the disease and develop remedies. Certain cancers are easier to put into remission than others. A few can be cured. Some grow slowly. But we have much to learn, many trials to attempt, and unfortunately, many failures to grieve.

Victory over cancer requires follow-up clinical visits, additional treatments, a bit of hope, a bit of luck and prayer. It's a lot of hard work, and no one gets a trophy. This is especially true of AML.

My football analogies provided a means of communicating progress, or a lack thereof. Moving the ball closer to the goal line gave encouragement to me and those following my journey. And though I announced scoring a touchdown with my completed stem cell transplant, the game did not end.

Now, twenty-one months later, I feel normal again. I have learned to recognize, and have not experienced, reduced hemoglobin (a significant loss of energy). And since my injuries heal rapidly, like those of a normal person, my white blood cells are doing their job.

But things change. After my two-year anniversary in February 2024, long-term survival becomes a reality with acceptable results from a final biopsy.

Guest versus host disease, however, is a threat for the remainder of my life. Stem cell transplant recipients live in that reality. I am alert to its symptoms. An achy stomach or cough can be minor irritations or the onset of a serious issue with GVHD.

The result is a game with no ending. Patients and survivors carry on with a new normal. Life changes… forever.

But, for now, I will maintain that I have beaten AML. I am winning the physical battle so far, and the mental struggle is well under control.

It has been over two years since my diagnosis. And I can say I have achieved my goal of quality life. Scrolling through family texts to find the original date of my diagnosis, I enjoyed messages and pictures of the life we lived these two wonderful years. No doubt, we spent hours and hours, days upon days, in and out of hospitals and clinics. But I am struck by how our family achieved an extraordinary degree of quality life.

We patients and survivors must continue to move the ball toward the goal line. Remember, a cancer victim is a statistic of 'One.'

The volumes of data available can be confusing, frustrating, and scary. But those numbers do not represent each person. Everyone's response to the treatments is different.

People sometimes defeat the deadliest cancers. Some say I am a walking miracle. Well, access to the extraordinary oncologists and stem cell transplant professionals seems like a supernatural occurrence. And the support and prayers of family and friends certainly qualify as a miracle. Time will tell if this hard work, this miraculous effort, will provide a long-term, quality life. I've had an amazing start.

My best wishes to each of you.

Feel free to contact me if you have questions or just want to visit. Leave a phone number and I will give you a call.

William D. Bramlett
bramlettbooks.com
wdb@bramlettbooks.com

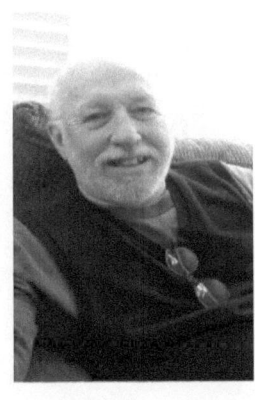

About the Author

William D. Bramlett is a pen name. The writer grew up in the southeastern U.S. and lives in Minnesota. An author of historical fiction, his characters and subjects are born from a love of history along with extensive travels throughout nearly every continent on the globe. A lifelong student of history and geography, he is also a dedicated outdoorsman who loves dogs, golf, and watching birds.

Other books include *Shorty, Rose Mountain, The King's Feast Series* and a children's picture book, *Robert Feller and the Lion Bully.*

William D. Bramlett
bramlettbooks.com
wdb@bramlettbooks.com